Blue Jay -

Overcoming Breast Cancer

Kaye Howarth

Published by Cook Communication

1407 Getzelman Drive

Elgin, IL 60123

www.author-me.com

Not affiliated with Cook Communication Ministries

Photos courtesy of Kaye Howarth

National Library of USA Cataloguing in Publication

ISBN
978-1-312-74923-8
Imprint: Lulu.com

Printed and bound in the USA

10 9 8 7 6 5 4 3 2 1

Dedication

To Eileen C. Cook, R.N. (Aug 12, 1941 – December 11, 2012, late wife of the publisher) who went bald as she endured brain cancer.

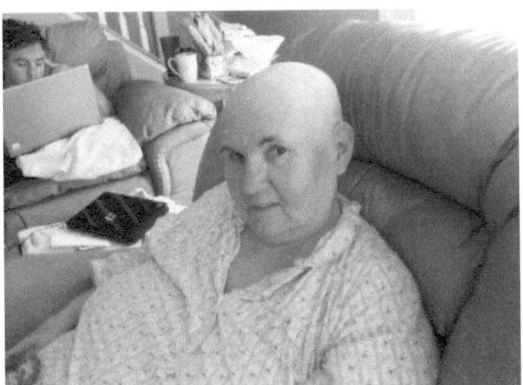

Kaye Howarth   Blue Jay – Overcoming Breast Cancer

Table of Contents

<u>My last Summer with two boobs-1999</u>

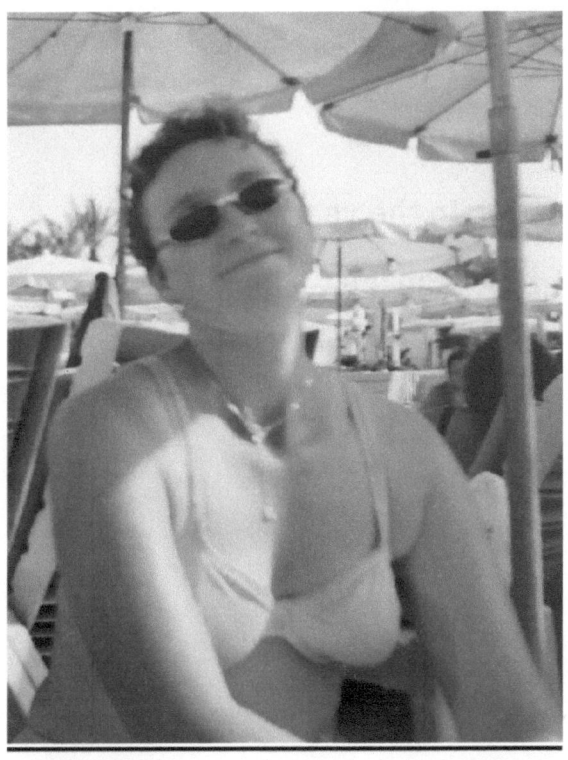

Introduction - Ripples

Daily Thoughts - "Why Me?"

Wormhole song in my ear~

~Let's all meet up in the year 2000.

My promise: "I will if I'm still here."

This book initially started life as a journal when my world was suddenly turned upside-down and inside-out, with an unexpected diagnosis of breast cancer. With such a diagnosis comes reflection on the life you have lived, and you wonder if indeed it could have been caused by:

- Lifestyle-Trauma

- Diet

- Stress

- Environment

- Poverty (does this really have bearing in contracting cancer?)

The reason I mention this is that there is an ongoing debate as to the cause of breast cancer. So, I would like to share with you my past, present and future lives to see if indeed my diagnosis was brought on by environment/Stress/and the life we led.

Let me introduce myself - my name is Kaye Howarth. The year is 1999.

This is my story, about my past, the present, hopefully a future. I am thirty-three years young.

I work part-time as a registered childminder, working up to the maximum hours you are legally allowed to work if claiming Welfare Benefits to top us up.

 Planning for our future once my children are both in school and I can go back to work full time, am studying for a "Diploma in Welfare," one day a week at our local Weymouth College, I do my course work once the children are warm and snug tucked up in bed.

Where I Live

My little family is lucky enough to have been given a decent divorce settlement from my ex-husband, enabling us to buy a newly built two-bedroom house with a handkerchief-pocket fenced-in garden and shed. This is in Broadway. where we lived directly under Pilon's for three years .When you walked beneath the power lines in rainy weather using an umbrella, sparks flew between the metal spokes.

Littlemoor Housing Estate is just across the road. It's don't-leave- your-keys-in-the-car country. Weymouth.

Eventually we have to sell our two-bedroom house in Electric City, Emily needs her own bedroom, having reached the grand age of seven, while George is three.

After much property searching every weekend, we decide Portland island is the place for us, mainly due to the house prices. we fall in love with a terraced house in Grosvenor Rd, Portland, Dorset.

Our little two bed house is quickly sold. Packing, and moving days, key exchanges arranged, we are set to go.

We set off for our Removal van for our new life in Portland.

But this wasn't to be straight forward. As we drove across the causeway, singing happily along to the children's yellow tape of nursery rhymes, the traffic slowed down to a crawl - to a long traffic jam.

Military Police were walking down to each car, leaning in to talk to the driver, explaining a problem.

You really couldn't make this up - the Island was having to be evacuated.

Evacuate! -1940's World war bomb Found!

We were allowed to go onto the island for an hour-to drop off our things in the van, but then everyone had to vacate-

Emergency accommodation had been arranged at all the Caravan sites in Weymouth whilst the Bomb Disposal Unit took care of the bomb.

Hopefully, our new home won't be blown up.

We chose to stay at Mum's! We did miss some good parties that weekend apparently!

Happily, the bomb was deployed safely and two days later Portland folk were given the all-clear to return home.

This has become our world - living on a small island, surrounded by the sea, and Portland Working Stone Quarries. Five minutes down the road is Easton square -a lovely park, and shops that covered all your needs, even a Butcher's.

On weekends we take regular walks out on the headland to visit Portland Bill. The cliff walks there are breathtakingly stunning as you look out to sea watching the White Horses, and hear the powerful waves crash up against the Jurassic rocks. You look up to the alternating colours of the sky in response to hearing the cries of airborne seagulls, effortlessly gliding in the pink, mauve skies of winter (or clear blue of Summer, depending on the season). This is where the sea hammers, and the children can let off steam. Pulpit Rocks are to your right as you walk round the Red and White Lighthouse-Portland Bill. The coast path leads you to the old "Red Crane," further along the path, down the cliffs that still stand strong.

Often Mum would drive over from Weymouth & come too, usually ladened with bags of food shopping to help us out. After paying the interest on the mortgage we were left with only £7.50 a week for food.

"Chesil beach Causeway," is the only road on and off the island. In stormy weather or heavy snow, the 'Causeway' floods and it becomes impassable. Portland becomes completely cut off from Weymouth - the next town -and the rest of the world. Hey – this is bliss!

Here we live the dream in our spacious three-bedroomed home with stoned terrace in Grosvenor Road, with a mortgage and a menagerie of two rabbits. Molly is a big grey long haired fluff ball rabbit. Toby, white and short-haired, was saved recently from the local pet shop where nobody wanted him due to some neurological deficiency. It caused him a head-banging motion, The rabbits gain comfort from our old cat "Pickles," who on windy rainy days would get into the open rabbit hutch, giving them free reign to hop in and out into the garden.

Pickles is always welcome in their warm straw hutch, where they all snuggle up companionably.

My Story, My Therapy

My first book **Bald Bird - My Story of Surviving Breast Cancer-** began life as

"Our Journey through Cancer Journal,"

My Cancer Nurse suggests keeping a journal therapeutic. helpful to record the rollercoaster ride, that we have been thrown on - or under.

Every night, having written in my journal, I lay my pen down, and pray so damned hard with God to just let me see my children get through school. I was greedily pushing my luck, but I still would pray harder for more... *Let me see them get to college.... Please God!*

Now that was twenty-three years ago, and I never thought I would be so lucky as to watch not only my children grow into adulthood but am given the gift to not only meet my grandchildren I am blessed to be able to watch them grow up too.

I have been supported by the most fantastic surgeon and breast cancer team, GPs, family, and colleagues.

Looking back to the causes that may have triggered my cancer could have been living in electric city; we lived there for three years. At that same time, five young women within three miles were also diagnosed with breast cancer at the same time as me.

Stress, alcohol, and lifestyle have also been a strong in-dicator, effecting my body, mind, and soul, and I would like to tell you about this as honestly as I can.

Past Ripples

<u>1965</u>

In 1965, Mum was a young, naïve, seventeen-year-old country girl. A young Audrey Hepburn lookalike, she was beautiful - stunning actually – who, unfortunately, caught the eye of a local farmer from a neighbouring farm.

 A man of twenty-seven, tall. dark and very handsome, working as a manager for a mass turkey producer and rare chicken breeds. He frequently travelled abroad, repping for the company for contracts,

He - Dad had recently separated from his wife with two young daughters (I now know why). Dad had a fancy sports car and, when he and Mum began dating, he would pick her up on a Sunday morning, and drive her at nail-biting speed, a cigarette between his lips, to Norwich City - just for a coffee. It was so exciting -film star stuff to a country girl-like Mum.

Mum did feel like a film star, with her headscarf on and the wind blowing through her hair, as they raced and weaved through the Norfolk countryside. She fell in love with him, and he her - a new lifestyle was opening up for her. Our Grandad didn't like him, didn't trust him... He thought something was off and he told Mum. Grandad also knew he already had a family and was legally still married. This created a terrible atmosphere whenever Mum went out on a date with him. Anyway, long story short - in November Mum got pregnant with me.

So, Mum faced being a single parent. Back then this was looked down on, and an embarrassment for my church going Grandparents. Although loving, understandably, they weren't impressed,

Grandma had already just raised her own three children and didn't have the energy, or the money to have a baby around the place, she was still working fulltime, as was Grandad.

Grandma knew of a Nurse/Nanny in the next village so, a few days after I was born, I was taken from my Mum & placed with Nanny Collison. Other children were there too, though of various ages and, sadly, I have no memory of them at all.

Mum had to get a job to support my payment for Care. She stayed in digs during the week in Norwich City, where she worked as a secretary, coming home to Gran and Grandad

On the weekend, Mum would cycle three miles to see me. She did this every weekend. If I were asleep in my pram, Nanny wouldn't let her pick me up.

This was heart-breaking for both of us.

1968 - Stress

Dad and mum then left not only Norfolk ,but me too.

They travelled extensively through Europe for the next two and a half years.

I remained with Nanny Collison.

Dad divorced his second wife, and they came back to pick me up-

I was then two-and-a-half years-old. We all drove off into the sunset-well Norwich City to the Registry Office and my Mum and Dad got married.

No one else was there.

After we set off travelling on to Dads new job, to go through what was then the 'Iron Curtain' - Hungary & Yugoslavia as it was called in the sixties. We were travelling, always travelling.

Dad worked away a lot - leaving us alone in some foreign country or another to fend for ourselves, and coming home with yet another love bite, after yet another conference.

Finally, Mum had had enough, she packed us up - booked on the next available flight home - and we went to stay with Gran and Grandad in Norfolk. Dad followed us shortly after, with his tail between his legs, begging Mum to take him back.

Mum loved him and took him back.

That was when my own nightmare began.

Dad began to sexually abuse me whenever Mum went out shopping. Taking me out in his Sportscar, parking in the empty house next door, he would conduct his deviant acts.

After he would ask me to put a cigarette in my mouth and light it for him. I felt especially important and grown up. All I remember was that he caringly had a pot of petroleum jelly in his dashboard to make sure I didn't get sore down there, . I never knew when or where these occasions would happen, I was terrified at night at the creak of the stair tread.

Stress

Living under these conditions was terrifying. I knew something wasn't right, but Dad would bring home a puppy for me and all was forgotten. Until the next time.

I prefer animals to people, this is where it comes from.

Four years later, Mum heard me whispering to my best friend as we played behind the settee about Daddy's 'Tickling Game.' Mum's friend lived down our road and her husband was in the

C.I.D. She immediately went down to her friend, who rang her husband at work. Then, as my dad came home later that evening, he was arrested.

Our lifestyle changed drastically, and we moved into a next-door bungalow, renting a room. Mum worked two cleaning jobs to keep us afloat. She refused to sign on-to take benefits.

Alcohol

Mum started going to church again shortly after Dad's arrest. She became friends with the local Vicar.

Now I was seven years old. Just up the road from us was an old Vicarage, and Mum and her friend Gill went to a Fete there. Sparkling glasses full of bubbly drink were standing around, and whilst Mum was chatting to the Vicar, I went around taking sips. It made me feel really happy-floaty and people laughed at me when I started messing around. Mum and Gill walked me home where I staggered about, pointing out a jogger, calling him "Daffy Duck," to which my Mum and her friend couldn't help but laugh. I liked alcohol a lot. It made me happy, and my Mum smiled.

As teenagers we all smoked and drank. We would go down to the local park, pinching drink from our parents' stash, hiding it in bushes - getting other teenagers to buy us fags from the local newsagents.

I found escape in alcohol.

Diet

Mum always gave us a balanced diet. Lots of salads and home cooked dinners.

Growing up- partying on weekends as a teenager continued into adulthood -drinking and nightclubbing, The culture in the 1980's was for women to drink as much as men, I had no problem with this. It was knowing when to stop was the problem.

Girl Power! I drank to forget.

I drank to get enough courage to go out of the door to join my friends. Drinking. Drink didn't Like me, but I loved the feeling it gave me. Nights turned out badly and the hangovers even worse.

As a single parent, every six weeks Mum would have the children over night for me - I drank and partied heavily with the best of them. On weekends I couldn't go out and I would put the children to bed and drink alone.

Mentally, I struggled with the outfall of my dad's behavior for decades. I didn't have the coping strategies to make sense of my past life, which in turn caused me to be introverted. I was angry with no real outlet apart from alcohol. I was exhausted from being a single parent with only my poor Mum for support us, and she worked full time herself.

Still, I did my best.

Bald Bird - My Story of Surviving Breast Cancer

Present-1999

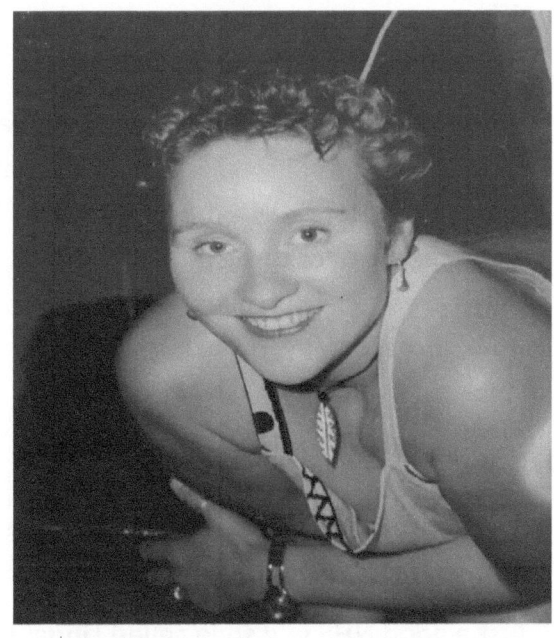

I am
thirty-
three
years
young.

Height 5.5ft, slimmish...was a Strawberry Blonde. I do still have hazel eyes. Divorced for eleven years, and a single Mum to my two gorgeous children Emily and George, both of whom are red heads!

Our family includes a toothless- tortoiseshell cat called Pickles, she dribbles incessantly (she's fourteen now) two rabbits, and two guinea pigs.

I work part-time as a "Speech and Language Therapy Assistant," at Dorchester County Hospital on the Adult Stroke unit, Hardy Ward. I love my job. Fifteen hours a week; spread over three days, my old unreliable car stoically takes me from Portland to Dorchester and back again, occasionally breaking down on Ridgeway Hill, which isn't fun.

However, that's the least of my worries.

I am at the moment on sick leave.

At present a "Bald bird," no hair.

Just a good NHS wig style called Linda. I don't wear this locally, just a woolly hat. On brave days I don't bother to wear anything on me head - my neighbours hail me in the street as "Sinead," which is as in O'Conner, the singer.

I don't mind.... I'm bald.

I found a Breast Lump, I have Cancer. I'm scared.

Cancer makes me revaluate my life.

Never before have I appreciated so much, the sweet (sometimes not-so-sweet) smell of my children's skin.

Kaye Howarth   Blue Jay – Overcoming Breast Cancer

I have been given a lesson to appreciate the day I'm in.
This is something I never really did before, usually planning years ahead.

A letter for Bert

I am beginning to have a relationship with my new lump. My fingers have taken on an obsession. Just like a jealous partner, they keep checking that you're there.

Of course, you're still there, aren't you, Bert? One hopes that, as with an old boyfriend who's bugged the crap out of you, you have hopefully picked up the vibes that you are not wanted anymore.

But lump - you're still here. I shall call you "Breast Lump" Bert, seeing that we are now- attached through my left breast. Just you know this, though. Bert, I hate you, and I hate all you've put me through.

In a weird way, though, Bert, you have made me pull my life together, I appreciate the new insight you have given me into how precious my life is.

Never again will I take for granted the sweet smell of my children's skin. The warmth of a hug with my children, laughing with my mother on the phone, chuckling at naughty joke emails sent by my best friend Annie, or the human kindness of the people who surround me. **So, Bert, it's just you and me, let the battle begin**

Kaye Howarth   Blue Jay – Overcoming Breast Cancer

A Definite Lump

My heart begins to pump so fast; I think it will explode through my ribs.

Whistling sounds ring in my ears. The bath I sit in has no warming for me. The bathroom walls zoom in.

"No God Please...not me!"

My hand moves around my left breast, I'm physically shaking. My breath leaves my body in rapid bursts. I feel I will pass out. My stomach constricts.

I mentally order myself to explore the outer perimeter of my left breast, once more.

There is definitely a pea-size lump.

"You bastard! You are a bloody shitty bastard!" Life I meant. I had only just gotten my life in order, at the age of thirty-two. And then you bugger me if this doesn't turn round and you kick me in the teeth, just as I start to relax.

It's funny, but at that moment my life flashes before my eyes, photographic form.

Snap! Me as a baby, lying in a huge pram, merrily sucking on my toes (no chance of that nowadays), oblivious to the surrounding wood pigeons cooing, and the glorious sunshine in the cloudless blue sky.

Kaye Howarth   Blue Jay – Overcoming Breast Cancer

Snap! Mum and I, now I'm a gawky, skinny teenager,
with stupid bunches sticking out of strawberry blonde

hair, standing on top of some hill in Torquay, with a parrot (the photographers) glaring menacingly into my trusting eyes.

Snap! Karyn, my best friend, and I - both hormonally charged sixteen-year-olds, at a local photo booth, pulling faces, rushing out after being blinded by the flash of a bulb. Waiting the unendurable three-minute wait for the four pictures to slide down the slot, self-conscious now, of the people guaranteed to turn up right behind you as the photos slide down....

Snap! First love Barry, motorcyclist, had a Moto Guzzi 50cc. Later he had a sporty three-wheeler car, orange and black, had to push to start it one time...

Snap! First husband, Weymouth Registry Office, children later, Emily first, then George, both inheriting my red hair.

––––––––––––––––––––––––––

Photos post-divorce

The kids and I in our new house, new friends, the children's, and mine. Parties, first days at school, crisp new uniforms...Christmases, learning the skills of balance on first bikes.

My wonderful grandparents Betty and Lesley, celebrating their 45th Wedding Anniversary. Photo with a Bouquet! Sob!

AM I GOING TO DIE?

Mum

It's at times like these that I thank God I have a fantastic relationship with my Mum. Once the children were in bed, bribed with various goodies to help them on their way (as all good mothers know how to support a child free zone), I dial my mother's phone number.

Now my Mum is a real character; she is classy, funny and has an inner strength that I have never met before or am likely to meet again. She raised me alone from a young and tender age, and it was a struggle for her, but she did it!

"Hello!" sang a happy female voice. "Hi Mum…" sniff…sob….

"Okay Hun…wot's up then?" she asks, her voice soft.

Sob. Sniff… "Hi Mum, I've got another lump!" (I had had an earlier lump, which turned out to be a cyst, aspirated 12 months ago.) Sniff…sob….

I then spent the next hour on the phone, with her telling me to make the doctor's appointment the following morning. I said I would. She said she would pay for me to go private if necessary.

Kaye Howarth   Blue Jay – Overcoming Breast Cancer

We end the conversation with her making me laugh. I can't remember what she said, but it did the trick for the moment.

Mum says all will be ok. Like a good girl, I believe her, Mums don't lie about such things. She says we had covered this ground before with the cyst, and that was all ok. We say goodnight and, after promising to phone her tomorrow evening, having made the GP appointment, we would catch up & see what the next steps would be.

I replace the receiver slowly.

The following morning, I give breakfast to bleary-eyed children. I Pack lunch boxes and fill juice bottles to the brim. I retrieve a Gym Kit from the airing cupboard for George. The children feed rabbits, guinea pigs, and toothless cat, Pickles.

I wave goodbye to their burdened backpacks as they disappear slowly up the hill, merging with other backpacks of assorted sizes and colours.

It is 8.45am, I make coffee, and get pen and paper. I watch the news for ten minutes, and then pick up the phone and call the doctors. The receptionist listens to me and my symptoms. It is a Monday- normally you have to wait for an appointment unless of course your leg is hanging half off. I am warmly surprised by the efficiency of the young receptionist who tells me to come in today at the end of Surgery."" Due to the circumstances Kaye, we would like to see you as soon as possible, so we will see you this evening," she says. This is a command I agree with.

The Appointment

"Kaye," the Nurse Practitioner calls me to her surgery. I sit down; give earlier medical history, including the aspiration of the cyst in the same breast, this time last year.

She smiles encouragingly, so I relax...a bit.

As asked, I now lie down on the examination couch, disrobed to my waist. (Once you have given birth, this is a ride in the park.)

The doctor gently examines both my breasts and confirms there is indeed a lump in my left breast. A referral is then made for the Breast Clinic, which is held at Dorchester Hospital held on Tuesdays and Thursdays. That's fourteen days' wait at the most for my referral appointment.

 God bless the NHS. She lets me get dressed in privacy, and when I leave wish's me gently, "Good luck!"

At home, Mum is waiting for me; I tell her all that was said.

Okay. I'll level with you. Inside my head at that moment I'm thinking, will I live to see my children grown? Have I got cancer? Is it in my hips? Bones? Liver? Kidneys, how much of my organs can they remove before the consultant says," That's all we can do for you?"

How do I keep myself and my family going until I receive my referral appointment? Patience just isn't my strong point, nor is relying on others for information, which is now what I have to do.

Waiting .Waiting. Worrying. Waiting.

Everyone sees me carrying on, whilst I write Christmas Cards (Christmas 1999),I send my children on various postage missions, and drink whisky (in moderation) in the evenings when the babes are safe asleep. to stop me thinking about "It."

."I wrap Christmas pressies.

It's funny, but as word of my predicament spreads around my street (although I hasten to add, I do not even feel ill, just run down), a support network begins to grow around me. These were friends I had lost contact with getting back in touch, telling me of various members who had pulled through...I drink in positivity.

Neighbours who are nodding acquaintances (due to busy work schedules, etc.) pop in with flowers, homemade biscuits for the kids, which are eaten quickly!" Homemade cakes come and Carol pops in from across the road for a coffee now and again. Offers of babysitting flood in, for as and when needed.

What do I tell the kids?

Throughout this emotional turbulent time, Ems and George are aware of my health. They are given minimal but honest bits of information, learning that I had a lump in my boob that needed checking out.

At this point, other family members stepped in, giving them support.

Emily carries on, being a teenager and acting hormonally. She hasn't quite reached the point womanhood yet but likes to keep up appearances. George continues with his Play Station Games, climbing and moving up levels with his lifelong friend Sean. Occasionally they can be seen on the fridge raids, raiding the kitchen for sustenance.

I spend the majority of the weekend with Mum, who is truly brilliant. She's so scatty and makes me and the children laugh. We eat loads and lay by her fire. The children start to bicker and argue...normality. Mum offers the children and me to spend the night with her. Emily & George are thrilled This is a wonderful treat that usually happens every other weekend. I choose to go home as I can only sleep properly in my own bed.

The phone rings. It's my Uncle Danny, quelling my ensuing fears of the up-and-coming appointment. We say goodbye.

The house at this moment feels very, very empty.

Working week and Supportive work colleagues

It is Monday, I go to work at Dorchester Hospital, and I have spoken with my boss (and friend) Natalie, the Speech Therapy Team Leader. (I'm lucky in working in the caring profession,).

She makes me a coffee; I gather my thoughts.

We sit down for a coffee with Claire, another Speech therapist in the office.

I tell them all that has happened. They are supportive, Natalie suggests it would be an idea for Claire to go with me to the appointment; I am relieved, truthfully...because...

1. Claire has breasts.
2. I can talk openly without fear of frightening her, and others at work.
3. I can tell them how shit scared I am really. Yes, please I say, and they give me a hug.

Claire and I then go to the Adult Stroke Unit to begin our day's work. As a word of advice to anyone who can manage this, work is a great distraction and anchorage, although intermittently thoughts muscled their way into my head, but I concentrated hard on my patients. I wondered what they would think if they knew what was going on in my life. Looking at other staff, I questioned myself as to who else could be going through an illness I didn't know about.

Natalie keeps in close contact with me, telling me she had informed the Head of the Department of my condition. Thanks Nat, you're a star for me, because sometimes just having to tell one more person can really do you in, especially at work.

Days tick away, work, children, washing, cooking.

I find through the ensuing days that I am beginning to have a relationship with my new lump. My fingers begin to take on an obsession. Just like a jealous partner, I keep checking that you're there...of course you're still there aren't you, Bert!

Seems like a lifetime.

Two weeks isn't really a long time, but it's like anything of such importance.

> Waiting for exam results, waiting for
>
> a reunion. it seems a lifetime.

Emily and George continue in their childhood. People continue with their everyday life, normality.

I'm jealous of their uncomplicated lives, don't they know I could be dying? Don't they know my children could be left without a mother?

I'm so angry at this blow life has given me.

I hate this life. I hate this, cancer. I love life and want to live forever. I want to see my children grow into adulthood. I want to see Emily and George graduate, go to the prom, college, to get married.

I want to have grandchildren sit on my knee. I bargain with God, "Please, God just give me ten years to see my children safely grown!"

> *I look down at the kitchen floor; Pickles our cat is meowing pitifully at my feet, looking up at me lovingly. She is noticing my emotional state, I then notice the cat flap has been locked. I want the cat not to have peed on the kitchen floor.*

Watching the letter box

I am not sleeping at all.

I'm getting grumpy with the children, and the entire universe. Busying myself over the next few days with all the household jobs. I'm trying hard to remain normal.

I go out and clean the rabbits in the howling, windy rain, and look up at the sky and shout… "Why me. What have I done!" My words are dragged out of my mouth and thrown away to the grey skies above.

Two sets of eyes look at me, with soft twitching noses.

Molly, a grey long-haired bunny, turns to Toby, a pure white rabbit. I rescued him from the local pet shop as no one wanted him; He sways like a head banger, (some neurological problem) with pink eyes, and ignores me. The Guinea pigs squeak and huddle in their straw, refusing to even acknowledge me - this strange noisy human. (They would, of course, be different if a carrot were involved, for it would be in their warm domestic hutch.)

I slop about with clean straw and hay, making them comfortable they do not want to come out today, although they have total freedom to run in the garden.

My hands are numb as I change the water feeders. What is my brain thinking about? "Cancer, the IT in my TIT," I think this and laugh to myself.

Kath, my elderly next-door neighbour is emptying her bins, shakes her head sadly at me. Kath must think I've finally lost it, I say this to has jumped into the rabbit hutch with Molly and Toby, who grumble, hiss, and cuddle up anyway.

I go inside to the kitchen. I need hot coffee to warm my frozen hands. Turning after flicking the kettle on, a large white letter drops through our letter box, silently landing on our "WELCOME" doormat.

This is the referral' I know it…It is, I'm right. Opening the letter with shaky hands, I read that I have an appointment in two weeks' time…and my consultant will be the same one who aspirated my cyst last year. I am lucky, he is brill.

I stand motionless with the letter in hands, in my green wellies, straw in hair, and cry.

The Referral

Having finished my work shift, I clamber down the hospital stairs. My energy level right now feels strangely low, and I feel totally drained. To keep my energy level up I have to eat every two hours, although eating makes my jaw ache, and I am finishing my meals long after everyone else.

I meet with Claire in our office. We discuss patient notes and ideas for helping patients, relevant information. Then we discuss what we did on the weekend, and various middle of the range chit chat.

The time has arrived for my appointment at the Breast Clinic. Claire and I gather ourselves. My heart begins to speed up.

"Are you sure you don't mind coming with me?" I'm now feeling apprehensive to say the least; I know Claire won't let me down, though I ask any way.

"Come on sweetie," Claire takes charge, and leads me to the door, downstairs across the passage, through another door. We have arrived. We turn right into the Breast Clinic.

The receptionist smiles warmly, acknowledging my name - firstly verbally - then checks out my NHS ID badge, which after sitting down I remove swiftly and put in my bag.

The Breast Clinic is fairly quiet. It is early - 1.45pm. at 2.00pm the clinic swells with women of all ages, partners, and children, including a few men patients. (This is not just a female disease, I remind myself.) Claire squeezes my hand reassuringly. I'm embarrassed as my palms are now damp and clammy; Claire doesn't seem to have noticed.

My name is called by a cuddly blonde nurse, Claire releases my hand and gives me a "keep your pecker up" wink.

I follow cuddly blonde nurse lady through to an Apricot room (meant to make the experience more relaxing), which has a chair and examination couch. I am asked to strip to the waist and put on a batman-like cape, I feel a bit of a prat, but do so.

My consultant (mine in the loosest connotation) he does make you feel like you are his only patient, ignoring the swelling number of patients outside my room. Mr. Consultant introduces me to Jean the Breast Care Nurse. We nod a friendly hello. He goes through my Case file and earlier notes of cyst.

The examination of "Bert" is very professional. Both breasts are checked, normal healthy side first to get a general map of how the tissue felt below, and then the other for signs of dimpling, puckering, discharge (were looked for and not found). However, "Bert" did me proud, showing his full figure.

Fluid is aspirated (a syringe used to draw fluid from my lump). I don't feel a thing, surprisingly.

This will now be sent to the lab for tests, I am told. The Breast Care Nurse smiles at me reassuringly throughout the process.

I can get dressed now.

Once clad, Mr. Consultant explains the sample will be sent to the lab and results will be back in three weeks' time. I should make an appointment to return then. I am given a card to tell this to the receptionist.

I say "Thank you! "And that I will see him then.

Claire stands up on seeing me, I'm still slightly red in the face. I make the previously mentioned appointment, leave the ward, and discuss what had happened.

I tell Claire "I wish they could just give me the results now; I would give them every penny I had."

Three weeks is an exceptionally long time to wait.

It's getting bigger.

Things calm down during the next couple of days; working, continue being a mother.

I lay in bed one evening; I run my hand over Bert...my stomach lunges. "It's getting bigger!"

I go back to the GP. My regular GP is unavailable. I see another. This GP offers to try aspirate - inserts fine needle to drain lump and take and use as a lab sample. He tries twice to no avail.

I say that is enough. The GP's face echoes my realisation. I Inform GP I will make an appointment with Breast Clinic. Should have gone back there in hindsight. I leave the surgery with inner sense of foreboding.

Anyway, that night after tucking up the cherubs, my breast begins to throb like hell. I give in & hit the kitchen for Paracetamol.

I take it every four hours.

Burn - burns - go away; come again another day.

It's midnight. I phone the Emergency G.P.I ring the doctors' number as the pain is now horrendous.

A sleepy doctor calmly tells me to continue with pain killers. However, he tells me I am taking too many.

Asks me if my stomach feels sore, it does, so he tells me the correct dosage I should now take. He recommends that I phone the Breast Clinic first thing.

Today is now Monday, Mr. Consultant isn't in Clinic, so I have to make an appointment for tomorrow.

Claire once again accompanies me to the clinic. Jean the Breast Nurse calls me into the side room, examines my breast that now holds a lump the size of an entrenched ping-pong ball.

I give Jean an update. She leaves the room to get a consultant, whom on further inspection of Bert recommends I attend a Mammogram, he writes this on a pink card ,the appointment date for this Thursday,

My consultant will also be attending that day, so will be able to see me afterward. Jean confirms this.

I dress. Tears course down my cheeks. Waves of pent up emotion course through me. I ask what the lump could be. The Consultant tells me gently that he wouldn't hazard a guess - not without the lab report and Mammogram.

Tears continue to pour uncontrollably down my face; Jean asks if I'm OK.

The Consultant replies, sardonically, "obviously not!" Jean offers me a hanky, goes, and books an appointment with Mr. Consultant's secretary, to coincide with the Mammogram appointment. I take the card and leave.

I join Claire. "They don't know what it is! I have to wait for the lab report," I explain.

Claire diplomatically takes charge, leads me to our office, and gives me hot coffee and chocolate biscuits, still a tearful sobbing wreck.

Claire had been a star; she has my eternal gratitude. I reach the car, get in somehow,

I drive home, imagining my funeral, my kids!

I nearly ram a shitty-coloured Metro up the arse. The driver, a woman, glares through her rear-view mirror, mouthing obscenities.

I give her the two-finger salute. Life is too short, and I laugh despite myself.

Somehow, I make the rest of the journey home safely, where I gabble out that they don't know what it is. My Childminder gives me a hug and diplomatically leaves.

Evening. Mum phones. Be positive she says.

"It's that naughty cyst again," she wishes. I had allowed her to pay for me to go privately, like last time. I say that the treatment I am getting with the NHS is superb, that the time difference would be no different. We continue discussing her move into the house opposite us - the Holiday House we fondly call it. I clean there on a regular basis during the summer.

Mum's house is currently a health risk due to a cracked, broken drain somewhere in the bowels of her dwelling. When sitting in her sitting room, having a cup of tea, it's similar to sitting in the public lav. I'm sure you can imagine.

Mum plans to live opposite of us for about two weeks. Actually, it turned out to be three months in all. The kids were ecstatic at having "Little Nanny" so close.

We said "goodbye, I love you." Funny how that has crept in, ending our recent phone conversations.

I go alone to the hospital for my Mammogram, etc.

I have now found the loneliest place on the planet, a small cubicle where I await the mammogram machine.

I wear a cape round my shoulders like a superhero, just wishing I had the super chest to go with the image. My boobs get their mug shots, I then go for an ultra-sound, they pour gel over my breast, just like a Pregnancy Scan. I now see my baby, Bert!

The Doctor puts her hand reassuringly on mine. Mr. Consultant sees the results.

I'm booked in for a "Lumpectomy" in three days' time. That will be the end of "Bert" I think to myself.

"Hahaha" giggles fate. That's what you think.

My journey and all the people in my life were about to ride an emotional roller coaster which would cover the next year.

Now I know where and what I'll be doing for the New Year's Eve for the year 2000, and I won't be meeting up with my friends.

Operation Lumpectomy

I pack my bag, nightie, towels, toothbrush, along with a photo of the children.

I kiss my Mum goodbye, and kiss the cherubs, smiling and cajoling them not to tie poor Nanny up for too long, blackmail etc. They laugh. wishing me good luck and saying see-you-soons.

Anyway, the operation goes well, and after I have the best-ever sleep (being total knackered), the nurses teased, saying I was like waking the dead. That evening I was asked if I wished to go home, heeding my mother's advice to stay in as long as I could and rest. I declined their offer, snuggling down in my warm bed. I felt totally cosseted and spoilt.

On checking my operation scar the next morning, I find a wider excision than expected. This raises issues in my mind, like why?

Nurse says to wait for the results, which will take fifteen days. An appointment is made for then. Mum arrives and escorts me home.

The kids go wild on my return. Emily promises they had been gentle with Little Nanny and then runs off, giggling with George.

Kaye Howarth   Blue Jay – Overcoming Breast Cancer

My entire extended family phones me during evening,
and also my friends.

Fifteen days later

I sit in the Breast Clinic. pretending to read a magazine. Jean the breast-care nurse flits here and there, coming over eventually and giving me a warm hug.

My name is then called by the Clinic Nurse; I go to the Consultation room. Mr. Consultant offers a seat after shaking our hands warmly. I'm slightly embarrassed as my hand is damp and clammy.

Mr. Consultant speaks. My heart pounds.

He's sorry to tell me that my so-called cyst was actually cancer - a malignant tumour. Stage 3 Ductal C+ T2 C, 3 NI ER Neg. The tumour had been completely removed. However, Mr. Consultant felt that the tumour was margin-line, and that for a better result it would be wise to remove the surrounding tissue.

Mr. Consultant spoke gently and kindly. (The above paragraph does not portray his absolute professionalism, which is due to my poor memory. I was in shock, which limits my memory of all the conversation, I would like to stress that I couldn't have been dealt with in a kinder way.

Mr. Consultant gently explains my options - that I can have a larger tissue area removed, or that a

mastectomy followed by immediate reconstruction was also a choice.

He also explained that, for them to fully diagnose me, lymph nodes would be removed and sampled (assessed), depending on how many nodes were affected, and this would help plan further treatment. Such as chemotherapy.

First, I want to know what a Stage Three meant.

"If it were a dog," I ask, "what breed would it be?"

"A Rottweiler," he explains, "although it is an aggressive Cancer, we have caught it early. When we have the results of your Lymph nodes, that will give us the full picture."

I say that I would rather have a Mastectomy, have it all taken away, my inner thoughts thinking that this would give less chance of re-occurrence. I realise that I had already chosen that before I had even walked through the door.

Mr. Consultant draws diagrams of different reconstruction techniques. I opt for the back Dorsal Muscle (the back muscle is brought round to the chest with its own blood supply and forms part of the breast) and Silicone implant. Later I have the possibility of a nipple tattoo.

"Please take a few days to think about it. When we

meet again, we can arrange the surgery date. I have free the 15th and the 22nd of December", he says, looking at me to gauge which date suits.

I say the 15th.

"Well, let's meet in two days, and book." Mr. Consultant stands as we say goodbye.

Jean gestures us to follow her and we go to her little room. All others are occupied. I picture women wailing and crying, throwing themselves on the floor in despair.

I think I have been given a death sentence at this point. I actually haven't, but that is how I felt just at that moment. Jean asks me to sit.

We do. I cry. Tears of sheer fear course down my face.

 Jean gives me space. She then talks . She explains the diagnosis, and that all was not doom or gloom. I was young and would recover quickly from the surgery. Jean thought I had made an excellent choice for surgery, and that she too would have taken that path.

Jean hands us leaflets that I can read later, about breast cancer diagnosis. In the back pages are support addresses and phone numbers. Mastectomy information on Silicone

Breast surgery, how safe Silicone is, etc.

I am shaking and feel that I'm now losing my grip, I tell Jean all my bottled-up feelings and fears. I can't sleep. I can't eat. I'm so scared. Jean suggests that I visit my GP, just for a short-term measure, to get some Anti-depressants just to take the pressure off a bit. (I do this, and it definitely got me through). I arrange an appointment time with Jean to see Mr. Consultant for two days' time.

Two days later the date for surgery is set for the 22nd of December 1999, and I do still opt for the Mastectomy.

> *I never in the world dreamed that my wish for the Millennium would be that I would live. I vowed that no lump (you, Bert), would rob me of my life. I loved my life, my family, and besides, we had a party to attend New Year's Eve, and we would be going! That I promised myself.*

Breaking the unwelcome news

You know, sometimes the hardest thing in life is telling unwelcome news to the ones you love. I was dreading it.

Having gotten the results of my Lumpectomy, I had no doubt that I had a fight on my hands, a mastectomy and then the possibility of chemotherapy afterwards.

Mum opened the door, and just by looking at my face knew all in the garden wasn't rosy. She bundled me in the door and held me close once we were seated on the settee. My wrenching sobs told her the results. Mum in her wisdom told me we weren't beat yet, and that things, were luckily, so luckily, still at the treatable stage. We did have a chance. Emotionally I'm shagged, knackered, and my brain hurts. Everything hurts.

The thought of dying - not seeing my children as adults - hurts, being forgotten and replaced really hurts!

Kathleen from next door pops in to see how things went. I tell her through sips of whisky (a small plus in this situation).

"Oh dear!" Kath looks weepy.

Mum tells her things aren't bad; we're being positive, she says. He thinks I don't notice the look he gives her.

Friends from over the road (number 24 - we're 27) come in, we all sit together, and I get hugged a lot. People glancing through the window must think we're having a wife-swapping party!

Eventually people leave. Emily my daughter comes in complaining of hunger pangs and we all laugh. Thank God for children. Whatever's going on, they keep normality.

I feed the kids, and then chat about my decision on having the Mastectomy followed by immediate reconstruction.

Mum says not to bother with the reconstruction as this a large operation in its own right. I say I'm only thirty-two, I love the beach, and want to get back to normal as quickly as possible. I understand where Mum was coming from, but I'm being offered a gift here, although reconstruction surgery has quite a long waiting list. Plus, when I had come round from surgery, not that much would be different.

Two days later I confirm this with Mr. Consultant. He clearly explains the surgical procedure. He draws diagrams, explaining the use of my back muscle to be brought round to my chest, plus silicone implant. Ten days in hospital.

My Mum has decided to take time off work, to be my and my children's carer. I tell this to Mr. Consultant. Surgery is set for 22.12.99 over the Christmas period.

Now it hits me that this is not what I planned for the Millennium.

I have a party to go to. God willing, I could still make it, I'd hate for us to miss Steve and Sharon's party, for their parties were legendary.

Ten days before the operation date, I pop into Dorchester Hospital to give medical background, etc. Everyone mentally prepares for the upcoming date of the Op. The kids and I continue going to Mum's across the road for healthy meals, scrummy teas, long walks. Life carries on.

I phone Natalie on Monday (she is my boss) and tell her the results. Natalie then phones her manager. This is extremely helpful and takes a load off my shoulders, as don't think I could get through the whole explanation without bursting into tears. Claire phones me that evening, giving me love from everyone at work. I receive cards from them in the following days.

I find that, emotionally, I'm really struggling. I feel really down. I visit my GP again, who suggests a short course of antidepressants just to see me through the next few weeks, month or so. I agree.

The next few weeks drag by. Antidepressants kick in, which make me feel a bit spacey and removed from reality. Without the tablets I become very down. I believe that my diagnosis can only lead to one outcome, cheerful or what?

All I can think about is "cancer." I read all leaflets concerning this subject, front and back, I even have a secret stash in the bathroom, in case I need a quick top-up of knowledge. My family pretend they don't know about my secret hoard. They watch sadly at my obsessive behaviour.

The Millennium is fast approaching. We wrap Christmas pressies, put up the decorations. Emily and George bicker, I burst into tears. I don't want my children arguing on what could be my last Christmas.

I continue going to work and we have the Christmas lunch combined with Becky's leaving bash, so the hospital canteen is transformed to a sparkling grotto. We toast Becky, wish her all the best in her new life in Australia complete with her Doctor Boyfriend Matt.

I will miss her; we have become close. I wonder as I hug my colleagues, wishing Merry Christmas, when will I return? Happy Christmas, cracking New Year, everyone!

Becky and I leave together. In the car park we give each other a big hug. A skinny builder walks by puffing on a roly, giving us a questionable eyebrow- raise.

We both laugh and go our separate ways.

At home we celebrate Christmas one week early, due to the fact I will be ensconced in a hospital bed on the real day. We hug and thank Nanny/Mum for our

wonderful pressies. My chest suppresses the hot an-
ger that I feel this very moment, fear - jealousy, that if
I might not be here for the next Christmas. How long
would it be before another woman takes my place in
their hearts, of those I love. Irrational fear, but that is
what I think.

Snowflakes start to fall and thicken. As we look out
later, the snow has settled so we all tog up and go for
a walk. The local playing field looks beautiful with the
freshly laid snow. We all do snow angels and build a
snow man.

A wonderful weekend

<u>Dear Diary, 22.12.99</u>

I pack once again. Mum looks after the children. On my leaving she gives me a big hug. The kids believe this to be the beginning of a rugby scrum, and pile on in.

Extricating myself, I bolt for the car. I listen to the Mavericks at full volume.

Arriving, I check in, am named, and numbered in the form of a wrist band. I Am given a swish electrical bed that could get into all sorts of positions.

Mr. Consultant arrives, greeting me warmly, and then asks me to undo my garments (curtains are drawn). He draws the intended surgical areas with a black marker. Once happy with this, he says I can get dressed again now. He asks if I have any concerns, surgical or otherwise. I ask him to just check under my armpit, I think I'm getting a swelling there (I am Paranoid) ...all is fine.

> **(Have you ever become obsessive? You know, like that disorder where you keep checking if you've left the gas on or, having gotten into bed, you think – "did I lock the door?" Well, you well know you have**

locked the door, but you still haul yourself out of that lovely warm bed, go down the cold stairs, and check.

Now, every nodule, tiny lump or bump that lies under my skin gets checked and checked again. I find new lumps that definitely weren't there yesterday. (Or were they?)

The Australian Anesthetist arrives, explaining that he will be checking me during op and post-operative for pain control. Will be managed by morphine injections. "Great!" I speak. "There is an upside to all this!" We both laugh. He leaves.

The Florist arrives at the same time as Karyn (S.A.L.T). Karyn leaves a Christmas Cacti and card at reception as she doesn't want to disturb me. The florist bares a bunch of the most beautiful white roses, courtesy of my mum,

I'm frightened. I cry.

I will now use a diary to track my wandering thoughts after my operation; I will write when next able.

Dear Diary, 23.12.99

I'm in an electrical bed. I can hear the rain beating on the windows. I take a look at my scars, two symmetrical, blue stitches like fishing nylon holding me together, a neat clean mound has replaced my breast, and I feel bruised.

I have no nipple. My armpit is numb. But I'm alive! Tubes drain my back and my newly constructed breast. Now I remember being wheeled to theatre. I fall asleep.

I remember waking in the night, shouting, Morphine is injected, and I sleep again.

Breakfast, painkillers, nurses give me a bed bath. What angels! I didn't feel humiliated as I thought I might, just mildly self-conscious. Now, sitting on the commode was a different thing! But needs must. I feel weak and wobbly.

Visitors pop in to see me: Anne from the Children's Centre, and also Jill.

Mum comes in soaked. She tells me that our central heating has packed up at home and we guess at the odds of resurrecting a plumber on Christmas Eve, Mum rushes off, forever the optimist for the hunt. God, she looks knackered.

Claire pokes her head round the door we have a laugh together. She goes. Later I fall asleep, unaware that the day has blended into night. I wake up alone.

> **Dear God, if you can hear me, I promise that from now on I will lead an exemplary life, if only you will let me live to see my children grown. Please, I will give back tenfold, please......I fall asleep.**

It was a Crappy night's sleep, full of nightmares. I dream of a blackbird which is flying at me, gets caught in my hair.... I can't pull it out. I wake up bolt upright, screaming, or so I think. A Nurse injects me in the thigh, and there is sleep, peaceful, full, heavy sleep.

Dear Diary, 24.12.99

Christmas eve! 8.00am.

I have a visitor. It was Mr. Consultant's surgical assistant, plus a nurse. I show him my new boob. He examines and drains three tubes that come from wounds - two in front and one behind. I think I must look like an Octopus. All tubes are working well. I wish I could have a bath. I feel sweaty, tired, and grumpy. However, I do wish the staff a Merry Christmas, and could they thank Mr. Consultant for my wonderfully constructed new boob. They say they will.

In the midst of this conversation, two lovely bouquets and a large teddy with a balloon attached appears around the curtain from my Gran & Grandad.

Emotion suddenly hits me from all the weeks before. It seems to burst out of me. I cry.

I have a new friend - the cleaner, I am the only patient on the ward, as all other patients have been discharged. So, we chat about this and that and she then carries on with her multitudes of duties. Then, with a cheery goodbye, she continues forth. The nurses are lovely and join me on their tea breaks.

Claire pops in and goes. I wonder in my mind - has the cancer gone, has the cancer gone? **Bert, do you miss me, I don't miss you.**

Mum comes in frozen to bits. We have a long cuddle.

Dear Diary, 65.12.99

Christmas Day, I have had a bath!

I have a new roommate who came in the middle of the night. (She had a suspected heart attack.)

Then comes Holy Communion. I meet the Vicar who I regularly see in passing on Hardy Ward where I work. He smiles a hello. Jane from occupational Therapy is playing the piano. Now it feels like Christmas - she sings Amazing Grace; I feel like I've been given mine!

Waiting for me are Mum, Ems, and George. They look shattered but open their pressies.

From George a candle with silver stars.

Ems gets a gorgeous angel in a beautiful card.

The children are restless, uncomfortable in their surroundings, and ask Mum to take them home, I feel really fed up as I really want them to stay longer.

Now I feel really sorry for myself, I snuggle down and go to sleep. I sleep.

When I wake again, my Mum is with me, I'm so pleased to see her it hurts.

Dear Diary, 70.12.99

Excellent night's sleep. Felt low yesterday. The ward nurses invite me into the staff room for mince pies and coffee. Bless 'em. Things like that make such a difference. I then get shown into a side room, which has a TV and a bed.

I can use that room if I want to.

9.00am. Ward round. Bare all. Dr. agrees that one drain is clear. I ask whether it can now be taken out. Oh, what joy! I hope it doesn't hurt too much. I'm such a coward where pain is concerned.

I'm given a Paracetamol (I know this is a Placebo effect!) in preparation for drain removal. Mum is here - phew! Hand holder, gas, and air on offer.

Half an hour later, inside the ward, I lay down, quivering slightly. "Deep breaths" says the nurse, so I do, and the strangest sensation follows as the plastic tube slides from under my skin and back muscle, out of my body. Wow! I feel slightly dizzy and scuttle off back to my ward as soon as the procedure is done.

Two tubes to go before freedom. Mum and I go to the TV room, where other patients and guests turn and look at me. I carry the bulbs that the tubes drain into in a material handbag. I hope they think I've got my knitting needles in there. I say a bubbly hello.

They all seem to relax.

Dear Diary, 27.12.99

Good night's sleep. My heart does somersaults as I see my grandparents, Aunty Steff, and my Mum walking through the wardroom door . You can never underestimate the power of good that a family visit does.

We chat for an hour, and then I'm suddenly very tired. Mum sees this and whisks everyone home. Hugs all round first, though.

I feel restless now that everyone's gone and I can't settle, even though I am tired. I get up slowly and cautiously minding my tubes, pick up my drain bags and wander down the ward... I come across leaflets by the ward door. The leaflets are on breast cancer.

I feel depressed on my victory over this horrendous disease. Stand and talk to the passing nurses. To bed now, for I really feel physically tired. Write diary first.

Night. Night. Write again tomorrow.

3.00am

I get woken up by an elderly lady being brought in, a lady in her sixties. She comes in to have her abdomen drained. It's ovarian cancer, she tells me positively. She's just come back from seeing her daughter in Australia for a final visit.

Sleep.

Ward round.

Drs say I can now have the other drains out. The first drain out is the one draining my front of my reconstructed breast. It slides out easily. The second pulls a bit, but all is fine.

Guess what the Dr then tells me......! YEP, I CAN BLOODY WELL GO HOME, I CAN GO HOME, ICAN GO HOME, HOME, HOME, HOME! BLOODY HELL HOME!

Mum pops in with Gran and Grandad, and Steff, looks thoroughly terrified when I tell her I can go home. Mum worries that I'm not worried, I get cross and tell her I'm so ready to go, Mum still feels it's too early.

Looking back, of course, I now see the overwhelming responsibility that Mum must have felt. She was worried that she might not be able to cope with looking after me and my whole household. My Grandparents have rented the holiday house in my street. They say they will help.

Kaye Howarth   **Blue Jay – Overcoming Breast Cancer**

Doctor comes round, explains follow-up treatment,
possibility of chemo, and plans to take the stitches out
after the tenth day, which will be New Year's Day then.
The Millennium, and the year 2000!

Please, I say, one day won't make any difference.
Could we do it for a day after? He laughs, following
my drift. 02.01.2000 is agreed upon for stitch removal.
I can go home tomorrow.

D-Day 28.12.99 I'm going home!

I can go home today!

Again, I had a crappy night's sleep although last night there was a late-night admission of a lady wearing an oxygen mask. The poor love rattled and wheezed all night.

12.15pm lunch, one of the nurses brings in her new fella, we laugh, and he goes shy.

Teatime and Mum at last arrives to take me home, I've been packed since 10.00am this morning. We give my flowers to remaining patients and give fresh flowers and cards to nurses. This seems such a small gesture for all the arduous work and dedication they have put into their work.

I feel like I've been let out of prison. Fresh, chilly air hits me. I feel shaky on the old pins. Luckily, Mum has parked the car close by wheelchair not needed.

I sit stunned through the journey home, feeling so relieved that part of my treatment is over. I can't wait to see Ems and George. I will make that New Year Party!

I arrive home to squeals of joy from my babies. We hug in the hallway. Eventually they let me go. I go through the hallway upstairs.

I feel disorientated as I put my things back in my bed-room .Mum has brought me a whole new fresh white cotton linen set for my bed. It is gorgeous. I feel tears in my eyes but push them back.

Mum comes over from across the street, gives me a gentle hug, trying not to squash my rebuild. Gran and Granddad are also there, with Aunty Steff.

I've missed my kids so much.

Once I'm settled, my visiting family say they're off but will be back again in the morning.

Go to bed early, finding it difficult to get comfortable. Now I'm not in my super-duper electric bed. I wriggle and huff and puff, making a triangle out of my pillows. I stare at the ceiling.

Dear Diary, 29.12.99

Where my back muscle used to be (now part of my breast), fluid begins to fill. This is really uncomfortable. I go to the hospital where Jean Breast Care Nurse drains it with a syringe. Ah bliss! I'm comfortable once more.

At home, watching, television I'm suddenly aware that every programme has women with bulging breasts. They have nipples jutting out, juggling in my face, taunting me. I storm off to bed.

I grizzle pathetically. I'm not feminine anymore.

You see, now, lying in this bed is a different person, physically, mentally, and spiritually.

I think change can be a good thing, it has certainly made me reassess our life. I lay still, thinking of all the good things I have in my life. You know, all the things you take for granted: a house, healthy children, a loving family, Pickles snuggles up to me and, slowly as the sky begins to get light, I drift off to seep.

I have decided not to write my diary daily now, as want to get on with daily living, just get on with family life.

Sleep comes easy.

Results of Lymph nodes

I get ready - be still oh beating heart - I have made the journey on automatic overdrive, arriving at Weymouth Hospital twenty minutes later. Unusually, I have no problem parking. I know this. I go through to reception and to the waiting area; sitting and waiting for my name to be called.

As if on cue, another speechie (slang for speech therapist) walks down the corridor towards us. We say "Hi, how are you?" All the time my eye is trained on the room which holds the answers to the next few years of my life...hopefully. Speechie picks this up, wishing me good luck and calls her patient who then follows her back to her therapy room.

My name is eventually called. (Not that the waiting time has been long; just seems that way.) Dr D introduces herself; she is an Oncologist. In other words, she checks the blood of cancer patients. "Have I had my results yet?" she asks.

"No," I say.

She tells me that I have had 19 Lymph nodes removed, and a minimal amount of cancer was found in one. That entire tumour was removed successfully; however, Chemotherapy would be necessary. FEC (I'm not swearing that is the correct name of the chemo treatment) - six cycles.

Or, that is, six sessions in layman's terms.

Dr D then introduced us to another Breast care Nurse and leaves us to chat about follow-up treatment.

I talk through my results. Were they good? Would I be, OK?

The nurse says the results were good, but she couldn't give me an outcome. I'm given leaflets and a form to claim for the cost of an NHS wig. This done, Mum and I drive off to Poole,

We find the wig shop.

Wig hunting can be hilarious, Mum tries on a curly short haired platinum blonde wig that looks so funny for she resembles a confused Rod Stewart. She swings in the chair, grinning profanely, and makes me and the Shop Assistant roar with laughter.

I buy a wig called "Linda." It is a red, sandy, colour, straight, and shoulder length. I sign the form, hand over my voucher, and then - still wearing the wig - I exit the shop. We are going to watch other people to see if they notice it's a wig or not!

I feel like a special agent undercover as we slip down the street and into the local supermarket, I'm scared the wig will slip. It feels hot and itchy, and I feel like I have a sign above my head. It seems to say: "Bald Bird wearing a wig."

I'm suddenly tired and need a drink.

We go hit a local café. Once we have coffee and cake, we find a quiet corner.

"Does it look real, Mum?" I pursue.

> "Yes, my darling you look gorgeous." We go home.

Jean the Breast Care Nurse phones, I give her my results. She says that's a fantastic result and couldn't be better. We arrange to meet Jean downstairs of the hospital on the 1st of February to look around Chemo Ward.

I show kids my wig, having removed it before pulling up home. George thrusts it on his head and we roar with laughter, for he looks just like his sister! We go to the holiday house for a coffee and to show Grandma and Grandad George in his wig.

Next Step

Today I go with Mum to see Jean the Breast Care Nurse. She gives me a warm hug. Mum asks various questions about the up-and-coming chemo and asks what we should expect.

Jean gives information on how the body reacts, how over the sessions one's immune system becomes weaker, so a wise move is to stay away from fluey people, or coughs and colds etc.

Jean then leads us to the Chemo Ward. We take things slowly as I tend to get breathless.

We stop momentarily for me to gather a second wind. I am then introduced to the nurses.

The room once again is a pretty peach colour, with rows of comfortable seats, just like any other waiting room, I don't know what I was expecting. We say goodbye to Jean and thank her for showing me around.

Mum drives us home. Thank you, Mum; you're a star.

Xxx

The Millennium! 2000!

Happy New Year everyone!

It is sufficient to say we all made the party along with Ems and George and our next-door neighbours Kath and Tony, all wandering up the street together.

I felt noticeably light and fragile.

Tony told me I looked beautiful in my long black and white dress. I looked at my reflection, and it is not the real me that stares back. I look into the hollow-eyed thin person. But I shrug and think, whatever, for I'm still here. Emily came up to bring me downstairs.

We go to the party.

> **I wonder if you can remember what you did for the Millennium. I know I will never forget.**
>
> **Happy New Year Everyone. Joie de vivre!**

First Chemo Session

Mum comes with me for the first chemo session. The nurse explains the procedure as I settle myself into a comfortable chair where the chemo is administrated. They will put a needle into a vein that will be linked to the chemotherapy treatment, FEC.

The drug is made up of three types of drug - each one will give a separate sensation.

1. I may feel the sensation of ants marching across my chest, forehead, and nasal area.

2. I may feel lightheaded (well, I've always been scatty...so!)

3. I may have a metallic taste in mouth.

Whilst this is being explained to me, I take in the other ladies. Some are wearing wigs, and some aren't. Some wear cold caps (supposed to stop your hair loss) and they are all at various stages of treatment.

One lady is being told that she can't have her final course of chemo today because her blood count is too low. She is really pissed off but takes it on the chin and re- appoints.

"How long does it take for the hair loss to start?" I ask.

About two sessions, I am told.

My friend Liz is getting married in two months, I wonder if I'll have hair. (Turns out I wore my wig Linda that day.)

I recognize a lady from the day of my positive diagnosis. She has waist-long, straight blonde hair, and her name is Jean. Before we start our first session, we swap phone numbers and book times to attend our second session together. We become allies thenceforth.

Mum leaves me with Jean and will return an hour later. Jean and I sit, get lined up, and chat. We take each other's mind off what we're doing. The treatment surges through our veins.

I do feel the ants crossing my forehead and chest. Mum arrives just as the Chemo finishes. I say goodbye to everyone. I say, "See you next time!"

Mum drives me home; I feel like crap and promptly burst into tears on Ridgeway Hill. Mick carries on driving me home.

It just isn't fair! What have I done to deserve this?

During that first week, I drink lots of water. Mum has brought me a water filter jug that is by the side of my bed. It is constantly refilled as I drink to flush out the toxins,

I am wiped out, no energy, and sleepy. I spend hours drifting in and out of sleep. Below our bedroom drones the daily hubbub of life, Mum cooks, washes, irons. I feel left out and useless.

Through the constant care (and the fabulous cooking skills of Mum), I rally daily each day, feeling a little stronger. I must be feeling better, I think to myself as daytime TV is boring me rigid.

I lay in bed, dreaming.

George and Emily love to cook, so we set about making a cake. We have a laugh measuring, mixing, and making a general mess. George and Ems divide the empty bowl to lick out the bowl after; we look at our work of art, which resembles a Frisbee.

2nd Chemo

Okay. Now my hair has started to fall out. As agreed, mum that evening gets out the hair clippers. I am given a number 2 crew cut. I have chosen this action, as hair falling out is distressing, so quick restyle is my solution. I now wear a woolly hat to cover the fact that I am truly "A bald Bird!"

<u>My Chemo appointment</u>.

Jan my fellow patient, is already there, and we look at each other and nod... "You too," we say, and we are now crew-cut twins. We go for our chemo; our respective other halves leave the ward together.

Dr D checks my blood to make sure I'm not anemic (or any other thing which could cause stop of treatment) and all is fine. I get my drugs...ants crawl up my nose and across my forehead.

I'm on a promise today. After treatment Mum and I are going to McDonald's for lunch. This is a hit, and always from now on it is a stop we will make. I tell Mum I'm going straight to bed this time, as trying to stay up doesn't pay dividends.

I crash. Mary Poppins alias Mum works her miracles in the kitchen. I get up and join my family for tea. I work (I don't have an appetite at present) through the wonderfully nutritious meal before me and I drink gallons of water. I try to make light conversation with all around me.

Then I have an almighty urge...... being toiletry for a minute and have to dash to the loo for a number 2. I haven't done that for what seems like an eternity. Ah bliss! I never thought I would so enjoy a poo. Exhausted from the excitement, I go to bed. (Also, I get wonderful stuff from doctors later that week: Lactulose, a blessing for the bound.)

Downstairs, Mum continues cooking, singing her God Songs at high decibels. She makes me chuckle as I lay in bed. She warbles away merrily to herself, and Ems and George are a captive audience. I doze off. Next thing I know it is dark. The house is quiet, and Pickles has curled up next to me.

 The mother of the washing, ironing, and comforter of children has gone to her own bed across the way. God Bless you Mum, how would I ever manage without you. Thank you for all your demanding work and never doubting spirit that supports mine when I'm doubting.

The following day we share with Mum and go over to the holiday house. We go for a short walk, and then have tea. We play board games and chill.

That night I go to bed mentally shattered. Putting on a brave face to the world is mentally exhausting.

In the morning I think I've found a lump in my right breast. I phone Jean Breast Care Nurse; she will check it for me after I've had my third Chemo. Here I go again, checking, checking...

Emily and George

Throughout my diagnosis, I have tried to be as honest as I could be without trying to frighten Ems and George too much. Emily has a firmer understanding of what we're going through and, bless her, has taken looking after her brother to heart.

It's difficult to keep normality going when such things as illness raises its head within a family, but I think it's important to keep a balance. Both Ems and George continue to go to school. However, I did phone both schools and inform them of my treatment and asked them to contact me if either child was finding it difficult to cope or was terribly upset.

Children can be strong, and some can be viciously cruel. George came home with a bruised face one day, I got out of him gently that a lad had teased him about me having no hair, "Cancer Mum," - so George retaliated, and they had a punch up in the school yard.

I went to the school the next day and waited for said boy, after school. Drawing him aside, I warned the little shit never to touch George or tease him again. I was so sodding angry, and he saw that. Needless to say, this never happened again, as far as I'm aware.

Something to Look Forward To!

Mum takes the kids swimming. Mum has taken out a membership at a hotel where there's a pool, with lots of rubber tubes floats, and toys.

Ems and George have hours of fun chasing Little Nanny as they call her around the pool, having play fights with the foam tubes.

Happy times and a safe way for them to let off steam!

My poor mother! Love you so much.

xxx

3rd Chemo, 15.03.00

Mum again drives me to Chemo. We see Jean about a lump in my right breast. Happily, she believes it to be hormonal. However, an appointment is made for a mammogram this Thursday. Dr D has also examined me and agrees.

I have chemo. Jan my Breast friend joins me. Now we both look like Army Recruits. The session finishes. We book the next session. Mum drives me home. However, we are low on food, so we decide to stop off at Asda to stock up. I am wearing a green woolly hat today. I couldn't be arsed with" Linda."

You know, I must be accepting my illness and preparing myself in some way for what would happen next. I was wandering round the veg aisle looking at food. I didn't really want to eat. And then wham!

"Hi Kaye, how are you?" Sean says.

Sean is the husband of Karen. Karen and I had our first-born children at the same hospital ward. We became firm friends, and found we lived in the same street. Eventually, I moved away from Dorchester to Portland, so we now just bump into each other now and when. But it's always such a treat to see them.

Anyway, he carries on teasing me. "Smart hat!" he jokes. I take a deep breath and say, "Haven't you heard?" I then calmly explain what has happened to me, about chemo and being bald.

He's great and asks me questions. Am I OK? Is there anything I need? He says he's sorry to hear that. "Me too, I say." Sean gives me a big hug. I send my love to his wife, and we say goodbye. It was just an average conversation in a shopping Isle. Mum rests her hand on my shoulder, gently smiles, puts her arm round my shoulder and leads me on to finish shopping.

Once home, I crash again, I'm knackered.

Mum, once again over the next five days, cooks, cares, loves. I'm knackered and look it, my skin looks grey, I am hollow-eyed, and I feel and look like a walking skeleton. I have lost lots of weight. I'm feeling low, too.

I Feel a bit sick on the journey for the mammogram, but somehow, we get there.

I am wearing "Linda" and feel a total prat. I'm now feeling very tearful and vulnerable, so I slope off up-stairs with Ems and George. George is on his Game boy we share. I mutter angrily to myself.

That night Emily is sick.

George wakes up crying with a raging earache, and a temperature of 102. He sleeps in with me, so I can keep an eye on him.

We're all worn out. In the morning, Mum gets Calpol. George rallies later that evening. It is a few days after that when poor Georgie feels well enough to return to school.

I see George off to school and decide that I will go into Weymouth. I will go to the library and get a delightful book to read. I park the car and walk through the town. I go to the library.

I find an awe-inspiring book, though deeply sad, of a young woman who had breast cancer. Her name was "Ruth Picardie", and the title was "Before I say Good-bye," I can only read a few chapters before tears are pouring down my face. This is a strange need in me, to find out how women my age cope, or try to cope, with this illness. Ruth did it with courage and that's what I need to know.

Just at that moment I have a terrible feeling, I don't think or can't remember getting a parking ticket... Shit. My memory (chemo brain) is really something at the moment. I leave the library bookless, tearstained, and in a panic.

I tank it past the art shop, and as I do so I see a painting by numbers picture of a Norfolk scene. The setting looks just like Burnham Overy Creek, which is where I was born, I have to have it, scrabble in my purse for the change (a £1.99 sheer bargain). I steam in - pay in seconds to a bemused gentleman – and then leg it to the car park.

Grabbing breath, I puff and pant to the car. Almost unable to look, I check to see if I did indeed get a parking ticket. Peering through one eye at my car window screen, I realize that I hadn't bought a ticket. (Crap). Even more surprising, (I have a Guardian Angel), I don't Have a yellow plastic wallet containing a car park fine!

Life is great!

Paranoid Thursday

I wait patiently at the breast clinic. I have become acclimatized to this clinic now and feel strangely reassured just being here.

I'm now in the Peachy room, having been called through for my check up and wearing the cape of Decency. Mr. Consultant enters the room. He checks my healthy side for the lump. But bless it, the lump has decided to do a hiding act, or hormonally disappeared. I go red and feel like a Pollack.

I have the ultrasound. This shows nothing.

I dress, leave, and drive home.

I recognize that an irrational fear has got hold of me. I need to talk this through with a professional, I keep thinking cancer is springing up inside my internal organs like mushrooms.

I phone my GP when I get in and he refers me to a counsellor:

> **Someone I can really talk to; someone I don't have to be brave in front of. Someone I can be honest with and say how truly frightened I am.**

Counselling Session

I now face a situation I'm uncomfortable with. I recognize that I really need support.

I'm going for my counselling session. Now, this is cute because I have done some training in counselling myself, but now have the tables turned and I'm on the receiving end.

I change clothes about eight times before I eventually get in my car and put on the stereo - fairly loud to cover my beating heart.

Once I arrive at my destination car park, I gently pull in and park u. To be honest, I consider doing a quick U Turn and going back out again.

 How wet am I. I decide to pull myself together and pull on my fetching, blue, floppy hat. I get out of the car assertively as possible and flop through the door and up go to the receptionist.

I give my name to Mrs. Smiley, the I'm-so-damn-happy receptionist lady, who sports a full head of hair (yes, I'm having a wonderful day today). She asks me to take the first door to my left and wait. I will be collected. I feel like an empty milk bottle. I flop (lack of energy, you understand, not bad posture) into a chair.

I hear chatter in the corridor as staff walks towards me. Oh no! I recognize one of the staff members and

pure, pathetic, survival techniques kick in (afterwards I can't believe I've done this). I grab a magazine and raise it high, in front of my face. I used to play netball with the staff member coming right past me. Eventually, I hear click-clack heels quieten and I get the courage to lower my magazine. There stands my female counsellor. Luckily, it's not the wing attack player for a team I can't remember the name of just at that moment.

"Kaye?" ...Counsellor Lady queries. "Yes!" I reply and follow her pink cardiganed back down a maze of corridors to her room.

Well, the session goes ok. I find it difficult to let go of my personnel barrier. This it has been my inner defense for years, but slowly I start to put out information.

Slowly I give my true feelings of how my life is right now, you know already. So, it's just to say it comes out in blips and blobs. My palms are sweaty by the end of the session.

My Counsellor suggests I look into getting a light hobby or an interest to take my mind off things. Meanwhile, she suggests I book another session for three weeks' time. This will be after my last chemo, as I'm really nervous about coming off of chemo. That will leave me without protection against my own cells that want to attack me.

I leave the building and sit motionless in my car feeling stunned with it all. I really need to do something to take my mind off things. We've always wanted a dog.

Aunty Steff Holds the Key

My Aunty Steff phones, and we chat that evening. She is thinking of getting a Terrier Puppy. Oh, I laugh. I would love a Basset Hound. I can remember Nana's Bassett Hound, low slung like a lion. Steff laughs, and jokingly offers to buy me one. So, we muse. How about a rescue dog, Steff suggests. This, of course, is the answer. Steff and I finish our phone call.

A few days later I receive a card with a Bassett on it and some money to buy a collar and lead.

Emily and I go to a local dog sanctuary in Poole. Sadly, no Bassets await us, although there are plenty of Heinz 57's and also numerous Greyhounds of all colours. We are the more sluggish side of the market. We are recommended to go through a specialist dog rescue, and I am put in touch with one such lady, Wendy.

She is in charge of Basset Rescue. She phones me that evening, talking firstly about my illness and whether this is a wise decision. She says these dogs are very therapeutic, and they make you smile. She also explained how they demand lots of work, Further, they are stubborn. Once the vetting process was discussed, she confirmed that a home visit would be arranged for Anne to do a home check with a breeder named Anne.

The following evening Anne rang us, asking if it was possible for her to pop round and do the home check, I agreed. Long story short - we were approved, much to Emily and George's excitement. On departure, Anne leaves us with some Basset books to examine.

A few days later Wendy phones us, saying there is a possibility of a male Bassett coming up for re-homing if we would be interested. I'm a bit knocked back as I didn't expect such a quick result and was planning to finish chemo first. However, having spoken with Mum, and children, we decide we would like to see him.

Emily and George stay with a friend, the thought process being that if the dog weren't a good fit, they would find it hard to leave him behind. Mum finds Wendy's house, and outside are a pack of Bassets which vary in size and colour. I spot a beauty. He's massive, but his tail doesn't stop wagging. Actually, that was Barney, the dog for re-homing!

Barney was soon ours having been signed, micro-chipped, gone through Eukenuba feed and ear drops. With a bit of help lifting his rear into the car, Barney was ours. Looking at him in the mirror with his ears blowing back looked like he was smiling. All that was needed to complete the look was goggles.

Home. Like a crocodile. Barney doesn't wait to be invited in. He hurtles past into the waiting arms -

squeals of delight - of Ems and George. They think he's great. As do we all.

Apart from the cat.

4th Chemo, 05.04.00

Following 4th Chemo, mum takes me home after asking if vitamin supplements are an innovative idea. The doctor is positive about this but says to be careful and not to overdo things. This had been a grueling session. Each session makes me feel weaker.

Mum sits for me in the evening so I can go out for a few hours. Luckily, the weather is still cold, and I can justify wearing a woolly hat.

5th Chemo, 03.05.00

I'm really pleased with my progress and am beginning.

to start planning things following chemo.

But my plans are thwarted- I wait for Dr Dean to give all clear for my blood check, before being allowed Chemo.

My blood count shows a high count of white blood cells, my red blood count is too low and unsafe for me to have treatment.

I remember that woman on my first appointment and I feel all her frustration. But hell, what can you do but just accept it.

This means I won't finish treatment until the end of May. My hair wouldn't start growing till middle of June… Hey, hang on here, I'm being optimistic!

I amaze myself. And with this I make my appointment and leave with Mum.

Mum suggests booking us a holiday. We walk slowly round the shops in Weymouth, I feel like an old lady in a young person's body. Thinking of laying on a warm beach sounds like heaven.

Staring in shop windows, we see a few deals and go in to ask for details. We then ask if the package entails health insurance. Insurance is something we can't travel without I remind Mum. This brings us down to

earth with a bang. It's £500.00 for a week. I say forget it, let's just go to Gould's Garden centre for a mooch round, tea, coffee, and some cake.

Sitting in the garden, I exhale and just enjoy not feeling sick or dizzy.

My last Chemo, 24.05.00

I have had my last chemo. I've done it. My families have done it. Yippee! I thank all the nurses for their never-ending support. Jean and I arrange to meet in six months and promise to stay connected by phone. We hug.

It's my last Chemo, I am so anxious.

Anxious to be not to be having more of these cancer cells busting wonder drugs, which cease my cells to develop in mad patterns, build, multiply and multiply.

I phone a Breast Buddy - A Breast Buddy is someone post treatment, who voluntarily links up with the NHS to support newly diagnosed patients.

My Buddy is Fran. She is two years post-treatment and lives just down the road on Portland. Fran knows and recognises my fears, concerns, and where I'm coming from.

Fran is calming. She tells me we are in charge of our bodies, that the chemo stays in our bodies for a long time, continuing its job of killing cancer cells. I would also be having three monthly check-ups for the first year, and mammograms yearly. Umm... I'm a little bit calmer now. We chat about our families, and then about my return to work.

Fran is now back to work full time. I'm planning to go back in September. Firstly, though, we have the children's six-week summer holiday. I will use this time to re- cooperate.

This is a clever idea, Fran says. "Don't rush back before you feel really well." We say goodbye and share good lucks.

Jean supports me, responding swiftly to any of my frequent panicky messages to when I find numerous lumps and bumps everywhere. In reality, these , have always been present, but due to my constant checks they are only now discovered.

I join the local Breast Care Support Group, as suggested by Jean. It is held in a church hall in Weymouth. A lady there had a Mastectomy twenty years ago. Also, there is a lady that has secondaries.... I also meet another lady called Mary. We become friends and arrange to meet. She had a Mastectomy five years ago. If anyone walked into this room now, they would question if they were in a keep fit class, the way people are so bubbly.

Getting back to life

The summer holidays fly by. We enjoy hot sunny days down at the beach, with picnics.

For me, searching out a shady spot, I am sporting a new swimming costume. The top is like a bikini sports top, covering down to my ribs. I am aware of the red scar on my back. My life scar, I have called it.

We build sandcastles and enjoy just being. George gets into an exceptionally large sand fight, mum has to intervene, as sun bathers are getting covered, those little sods. George comes back looking like a sandman. Ice cream is bought, and everyone settles back down.

Emily is making sand mermaids, using seaweed for hair. The sky is blue, and the sea gently laps. Life is good again; no life is brilliant. I look at my family and sigh contently.

The holidays are ending. My children have had a fun time just being. Family and friends spoil them. They seem strong little people now, for they are more in-dependent of me, more self-sufficient.

Mum is going back to work.

Back to work

Holidays are over, its September. School gates creak open, and swarms of children sway up the street on the path back to education. They pretend not to be happy about this as they chat excitedly with reunited friends that they have missed over the hols.

Emily and George have gone, the house is empty, apart from doggie Barney and me. I can even hear the mantle clock ticking. I sit and have a coffee, having tidied away.

Breakfast dishes done; I go upstairs to get my work shoes. I pause and look at my reflection; I wonder how my colleagues will react to my return. I have gained a little weight now, and my hair is now short and wavy. It's darker than my former Strawberry blonde locks.

I put Barney out in his kennel and that check he has clean water.

"Well Barney, this is it, I'm back to work!" I blurt out. Barney lays down on his blanket, looking at me quizzically. Walking back through the kitchen to the hall, I pick up the keys from their hook.

I stop, turn round, and take a last look. I thought this day would never come.

Driving to work I feel the rush of exhilaration.

I am away from home. I'm going to work!

Arriving in Dorchester, I drive around for five minutes, trying desperately to find a parking spot. (This is always difficult in a hospital car park). I have to give up and decide to try further afield. Cutting down the back streets, I turn into Dagmar Road. That is where I lived with my first husband - Emily, and George's Dad. Gosh, that seems a lifetime ago.

I park up, pause, and smile. I slip through the back alley to Williams Avenue and cross the main road. Before I go to the main hospital, I pop in and say hello to one of the secretaries in The Children's Centre.

After I walk up the steps towards the Pencils (a large mobile of different coloured pencils - some architect's dream), I turn left and get the lift up to Hardy Ward. I pass the large photos of staff.

"Hello, it's good to be back," I say quietly as I pass by.

Balloons are attached to our office door. I enter. "Welcome back!" banners are spread across the room and more balloons are attached to the walls. I see a card for me, signed from Natalie, Karyn, and Claire.

I turn then and get into my In-Tray.

Life slips to normality.

However, I find that, after a while, working in a hospital environment is challenging. I'm feeling a need to change direction workwise. I look into doing a Reflexology Course at the Weymouth College- a holistic course.

Ringing up, the course is 3 weeks in, but if I feel OK about it. They have one space. I pass the interview and grab the course! It's one day a week (perfect) and will fit in with my working hours. I'm proud of my dress whites, looking like someone from a Daz Advert. I have also decided that I definitely want to change my job.

I have always enjoyed working with the elderly and would like to go back to working in the community.

After many walks with Mum at Abbotsbury, along the beach path (where we always churned things over), we debate over whether I should or shouldn't give up my hospital job,

I decide to do just that. I have learnt such a lot in this job, and I will never forget the characters I have met. Especially my very first patient, Jimmy. Following his Stroke all he could say was the F word. But every Christmas Jimmy sent me a Christmas card.

Natalie and Karyn were sad that I was leaving but understood and wished me well in my new position with Carewey. I had gotten a job with an elderly lady and her son who lived six doors up from me. Things couldn't have worked out better.

Time ticks by and the children relax. Mum is well settled back to work.

Barney lolls around the house. Rabbits sunbathe in the garden. The cat Pickles, well, she's just the same, sneaking in with the guinea pigs.

We all regain our independence. I catch up with friends that found my illness difficult to cope with. Emily and George have as many friends round as we can pack in. I can recognise who's there by the trainers in the hall.

I relish not having to drive to work and I enjoy making new work friends.

I join "Bosom Buddies," a Support group and meet Monica, who lives on Portland just round the corner from me. She also works for "Weymouth and Portland Housing."

Monica asks if I would like to apply for a part-time cleaning post at Lady mead Hall.

I go for the interview but am offered not the cleaning job, but a Warden's position starting in February. It's all happening!

George chooses new colours for his bedroom, orange, and red!

Health check-ups pass well: 1 month, then 3 months.

Then it's Christmas. Mum cooks and we all celebrate. What a year!

Feb, March slip by. April, May, June and then July and, at last, I qualify as a reflexologist! Whoopee doo!

Now I work occasionally (voluntarily having got through the vetting process) as a reflexologist for Hamwick House, treating cancer patients. I work when needed. It's the least I can do. Now I can give something back to the NHS as a thank you for all the care I received.

Not the end!

2020

It's 2020 - I am completing this journal twenty years after being diagnosed with Grade 3 Breast Cancer.

I am now a grand fifty-seven years old, happily re-married to Andy ,living in Worcester, Worcestershire.

 Emily is married to Darren ,and working as a TA with Special needs children, and enrolled in university to become a qualified teacher and we have two beautiful grandchildren.

Mum is well and reliable as ever!

I have worked as a Support Worker for The Homeless with Drug, Alcohol & mental health issues at St Paul's Hostel for seven years. Taking a redundancy package to retrain as a Dog Groomer-Andy converted our garage into a Dog Grooming Salon & we established my own dog grooming salon – "Hair Off the Dawg!" - working from home.

George eventually moved up with us from Dorset, and now works at St Paul's Hostel as a Support Worker and is at University retraining to be a Counsellor.

I've rescued two donkeys from Ireland - George & Harvey, now re-habbed and happy in a local donkey sanctuary. I'm alive and well with no reoccurrence 20 years on from first being diagnosed with Grade 3 Breast Cancer.

I'm alive!

I never thought I would say this, but I have been so incredibly lucky. I have a loving family, Mum is Old Reliable, with my new soulmate Andy and children and now grandchildren.

Never, ever, be frightened to get help and support for breast cancer and after.

 I requested yearly mammograms rather than every three years, and the NHS supported me throughout. Still, I truly struggle with the fear of the disease returning.

Mental Health is important - I have continued to use and will always use/have the support of Counselling via my GP with anti-depressants,

For my past sexual abuse, I struggled, and still used alcohol to numb or cope with the memories. That just doesn't go away-eventually after a horrendous argument due to my drinking I joined AA-.Counselling for Sexual Abuse and GP support to help me begin my new journey.

And, of course, if I'm worried about any lump or bump, I still scuttle off swiftly and get it checked out by my GP! They are eternally patient with me.

My life has gone through massive lows and highs. It has been a rollercoaster ride of emotions.

I met and Married Andy, who is my soulmate, bringing to the fold his two sons. We have been married ten years this year. Thank you so much for your never-ending patience and support of me and our expanding family.

Andy is lovingly known as Grandy to our grandchildren.

George has recently bought his first house and lives with his much-wanted German Shepherd Nikolai (21st Birthday present) wahoo. So proud of you all my loves.

RIP —Barney, Pickles, and the Guinea pigs. We miss you still. RIP Charlie my Chocolate Springador dog, 9 years old (Shoe-pincher, and the lazy lump in my bed!).

Hello to Jack the Jack Russell and Pablo, a Chihuahua.

Hello to our new lives.

At last, our family is safe & free!

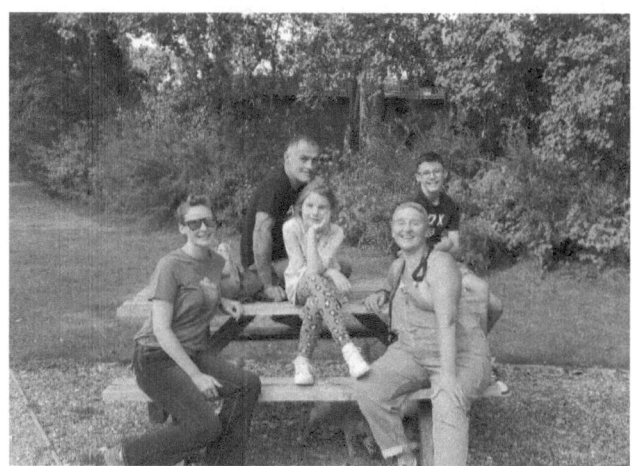

*The past events and environment I grew up in may have contributed to my diagnosis of breast cancer.

I & my whole family have had to carry the mind- numbing burden & shame, that Sexual abuse, causes. The aftereffects of living with the shame, stigma, and uncertainty of what was happening to me. Confusion in the fact I loved my dad but had to try and work out that this "game" of his wasn't right -

111

what he was doing to me – and later, find-ing out he also abused my little friends, which now makes sense as to why they stopped playing with me.

As an adult, the continual worry for my chil-dren in case Dad suddenly turned up - or one of my three other "Uncles "or an un-known member of his family that I didn't know may turn up unexpectedly to my chil-dren's school.

.Having to give my own daughter and son a photograph of my dad - teachers-at their schools to make sure they never ever went with him if he tried to collect them.

The constant fear and concern rippled down to the next generation to my daugh-ter's two children, my grandchildren.

The ripples from sexual abuse flow far and wide over the whole family not just the one child affected at that time, but the next generation and their little friends. My daughter had to let her husband's family know, too. The shame is continuous.

So now this stop. My Grandparents have now passed so has my father-I am not going to be ashamed anymore. I am telling our story.

We have done our time under the horrendous shadow of my Father - as have all my stepbrothers/sisters/and friends and my poor mother, who lost the love of her life, husband, partner.

Mum never remarried.

Thank You

Thankyous, where do I begin?

To Emily and George for all you went through, all your support love and cuddles, I love you forever.

To Mum - Old Reliable - Wow what a trooper for your never-ending care, love, and support. You were there for us as always. We love you so much.

To Gran and Grandad. We lost Grandad a few years ago and Grandma recently- we miss you dreadfully.

To Aunty Steff, Danny, Davina for all your phone calls and visits. Thank you.

Last, but by no means least, to my lovely new husband Andy, who I met at the Weymouth and Portland Housing Christmas Do, 2004. Andy, you mean so much to me. You light up my life with love, laughter, and kindness. We got married at Gretna Green on 31st July 2010. I love you so much, especially when your eyes twinkle!

I'm Alive!!!!!

To Dorchester County Hospital. Thank you for the gift of extended life.

To Mr. Consultant, Jean, all the nurses and all the wonderful women who I met along the way.

Thank you.

Kaye Howarth   Blue Jay – Overcoming Breast Cancer

To my Bosom Buddy friend Fran who sadly passed away.

To Monica, Bosom Buddy friends. We're doing well, aren't we!

xxxxxxx

www.ingramcontent.com/pod-product-compliance
Lightning Source LLC
Chambersburg PA
CBHW021829170526
45157CB00007B/2733